THE COMPLE
FAMILY (ᴜ
DEMENTIA

A Book for Dementia Patients
Caregivers, Getting a Hang with
Patient Aggression, and Dealing
with the Different Stages

Kate Spaull

Table of Content

INTRODUCTION TO DEMENTIA

Dementia is a neurological disorder that effects the cognitive function behaviour and memory of the affected. Specifically it is not a disease rather,it is a term used to describe the several symptoms associated with decline in mental abilities simply severe enough to affect ones daily life. Dementia is most commonly seen in older adults, although it can occur in younger individuals as well.

The most common cause of dementia is Alzheimer's disease, accounting for approximately 60-80% of cases. Other causes include vascular dementia, Lewy body dementia, frontotemporal dementia, and mixed dementia, which is a combination of different types. The specific symptoms and progression of dementia can vary depending on the underlying cause.

Memory loss is one of the hallmark symptoms of dementia. People with dementia may have difficulty remembering recent events, names, or familiar places. They may also experience challenges with language and communication, such as finding the right words or following a conversation. Additionally, individuals with dementia may struggle with problem-solving, decision-making, and organizing tasks. Changes in mood, personality, and behavior are also common.

As dementia progresses, individuals may require assistance with daily activities such as dressing, eating, and bathing. The condition can have a significant impact on the person's independence and quality of life. Dementia is a progressive disorder, meaning that symptoms worsen over time.

Diagnosis of dementia involves a comprehensive evaluation of a person's medical history, cognitive function, physical examination, and sometimes imaging tests such as brain scans. While there is currently no cure for most types of dementia, early diagnosis and appropriate management strategies can help improve the person's quality of life and slow down the progression of symptoms.

Treatment of dementia focuses on addressing the underlying causes and managing symptoms. This can involve medication, cognitive and behavioral therapies, and lifestyle modifications. Supportive care, including assistance with daily activities and a safe environment, is also essential.

Caring for someone with dementia can be challenging, both emotionally and physically. Family members and caregivers play a crucial role in providing support, ensuring safety, and maintaining the person's well-being. Support groups and community resources are available to assist caregivers in managing the demands of caring for someone with dementia.

CHAPTER 1: UNDERSTANDING DEMENTIA

Dementia is a complex and challenging syndrome that affects millions of individuals worldwide. As the population ages, the prevalence of dementia continues to rise, making it a pressing issue for healthcare professionals, caregivers, and society as a whole. This chapter delves into the multifaceted aspects of dementia, providing a comprehensive understanding of its causes, symptoms, diagnosis, and management strategies.

What is Dementia?

In this section, we will explore the definition of dementia and its various types and causes. Readers will gain insight into the underlying biological mechanisms that contribute to the development of dementia, including the role of protein deposits, vascular issues, and brain cell damage. By understanding the diverse causes of dementia, we can better comprehend the range of symptoms and challenges faced by individuals living with the condition.

Is Dementia Hereditry?

Yes, there can be a hereditary component to certain types of dementia. While most cases of dementia are not directly inherited, some forms have a genetic component that can increase the risk of developing the condition.

For example, in Alzheimer's disease, the most common form of dementia, there are certain genes that have been identified as risk factors. The most well-known genetic risk factor for late-onset Alzheimer's disease is the APOE gene. Variations of this gene, particularly the APOE ε4 allele, have been associated with an increased risk of developing Alzheimer's disease.

However, it's important to note that having a genetic risk factor does not guarantee the development of dementia. Many other factors, including lifestyle, environmental factors, and complex interactions between genes, contribute to the development of the disease.

It's also worth mentioning that there are some rarer forms of dementia, such as familial

Alzheimer's disease and certain types of frontotemporal dementia, that are directly caused by specific gene mutations and have a clear pattern of inheritance within families.

If there is a family history of dementia, particularly at a younger age or multiple affected relatives, it may be advisable to consult with a genetic counselor or healthcare professional with expertise in dementia to discuss any potential genetic risks and consider genetic testing if appropriate.

It's important to understand that even in cases where there is a genetic risk, lifestyle factors such as maintaining a healthy diet, engaging in regular physical and mental exercise, managing chronic conditions, and maintaining social connections can play a significant role in reducing the overall risk and promoting brain health.

Common Types of Dementia

Dementia is a term used to describe a group of symptoms that affect memory, thinking, and social abilities to the extent that it interferes with daily functioning. The several types of dementia are:

Alzheimer's disease: This is the most common type of dementia, accounting for 60-80% of cases. It is characterized by the accumulation of amyloid plaques and neurofibrillary tangles in the brain, leading to progressive cognitive decline.

Vascular dementia: This type of dementia results from reduced blood flow to the brain, usually due to a stroke or other vascular conditions. Symptoms can vary depending on the area of the brain affected, but they often include problems with memory, reasoning, and planning.

Lewy body dementia: Lewy body dementia is characterized by the presence of abnormal protein deposits called Lewy bodies in the brain. It shares similarities with both Alzheimer's disease and Parkinson's disease, as it can cause cognitive decline, visual hallucinations, and motor symptoms like tremors and stiffness.

Frontotemporal dementia (FTD): FTD is a group of disorders characterized by the degeneration of nerve cells in the frontal and temporal lobes of the brain. It can lead to changes in personality, behavior, and language, often before memory problems occur.

Parkinson's disease dementia: Although Parkinson's disease primarily affects movement, it can also cause dementia symptoms. People with Parkinson's disease dementia often experience cognitive decline, including problems with memory, attention, and executive function.

Mixed dementia: In some cases, individuals may have multiple types of dementia simultaneously. For example, a person may have both Alzheimer's disease and vascular dementia, leading to a combination of symptoms from both conditions.

Impact of Dementia on Individuals and Families

Dementia has a profound impact on both individuals and their families. The progressive nature of the disease and the cognitive decline it causes can significantly alter the lives of those affected. It's impact on individuals and families include:

Cognitive decline: Dementia leads to a decline in cognitive abilities, including memory loss, difficulty with problem-solving and decision-making, language problems, and reduced attention span. These cognitive impairments can make it challenging for individuals to carry out daily activities, maintain independence, and engage in meaningful social interactions.

Emotional and behavioral changes: Dementia can cause emotional and behavioral changes in individuals. They may experience mood swings, agitation, anxiety, depression, and irritability. These changes can be distressing for both the individuals with dementia and their family members, who may struggle to understand and cope with these new behaviors.

Caregiver burden: Family members often take on the role of caregivers for individuals with dementia. Providing care for a loved one with dementia can be physically, emotionally, and financially demanding. Caregivers may experience high levels of stress, fatigue, and burnout due to the constant responsibility of managing the care needs of the individual with dementia.

Changes in family dynamics: Dementia can disrupt family dynamics and relationships. The person with dementia may become dependent on family members for their daily needs, reversing traditional roles and causing strain on relationships. Siblings and other family members may also experience conflicts or differences in opinion regarding care decisions, financial matters, and long-term planning.

Social isolation: Dementia can lead to social isolation for both individuals and their families. The cognitive and behavioral changes associated with the disease may make it difficult for individuals to participate in social activities or maintain relationships. Families may also face challenges in participating in social events or outings due to the care needs of their loved one.

Financial impact: Dementia can have a significant financial impact on individuals and families. The cost of medical care, medications, in-home care services, and assisted living facilities can be substantial. Families may also face challenges in managing the individual's finances, ensuring legal and financial affairs are in order, and making decisions regarding long-term care options.

Grief and loss: Dementia is a progressive disease, and individuals with dementia and their families often experience grief and a sense of loss as the person's cognitive abilities and personality change over time. Family members may grieve the loss of the person they once knew and struggle with the emotional toll of witnessing the decline.

CHAPTER 2: RECOGNIZING SIGNS AND SYMPTOMS

The early identification and recognition of signs and symptoms associated with various health conditions are crucial for prompt intervention and optimal outcomes. This chapter focuses on the importance of recognizing the signs and symptoms of dementia, differentiating dementia from age-related memory loss, seeking medical evaluation and diagnosis. By understanding these indicators, healthcare professionals, caregivers, and individuals themselves can take proactive steps towards diagnosis, treatment, and support.

Early Warning Signs of Dementia

Recognizing the early warning signs of dementia is crucial for early diagnosis and intervention. While experiencing one or more of these signs does not necessarily mean a person has dementia, it is advisable to consult a healthcare professional for a proper evaluation. Beloe are some common early warning signs of dementia:

Memory loss: One of the most prominent early signs of dementia is memory loss. This includes forgetting recently learned information, important dates or events, repeatedly asking for the same information, and relying heavily on memory aids or family members to recall things.

Difficulty with problem-solving and planning: Dementia can affect a person's ability to solve problems and make plans. Tasks that once seemed routine or familiar, such as managing finances or following a recipe, may become increasingly challenging.

Language and communication problems: Individuals in the early stages of dementia may struggle with finding the right words, following or joining conversations, and expressing themselves clearly. They may experience difficulty remembering familiar words or substituting them with inappropriate ones.

Confusion and disorientation: Dementia can lead to confusion regarding time, place, and even personal identity. Someone with early-stage dementia may get lost in familiar surroundings, forget where they are or how they got there, and have difficulty remembering appointments or events.

Impaired judgment and decision-making: Individuals with early-stage dementia may exhibit poor judgment or impaired decision-making abilities. They may make unusual or risky choices, have difficulty following a plan or adhering to a schedule, and struggle with reasoning and logical thinking.

Changes in mood and personality: Dementia can cause notable shifts in mood and personality. Individuals may become increasingly irritable, anxious, or suspicious, and experience rapid mood swings. They may also withdraw from social activities or display apathy towards previously enjoyed hobbies or interests.

Difficulty completing familiar tasks: Individuals with early-stage dementia may find it challenging to perform familiar tasks or follow step-by-step instructions. Simple activities like cooking a meal, using a household appliance, or playing a familiar game may become more difficult or confusing.

Misplacing items and inability to retrace steps: People with early-stage dementia often misplace objects and struggle to retrace their steps to find them. They may put things in unusual places or accuse others of stealing their belongings.

Differentiating Dementia from Age-Related Memory Loss

Distinguishing between dementia and age-related memory loss is important as it helps individuals and healthcare professionals determine if further evaluation and intervention are necessary. While it is common for memory and cognitive abilities to change with age, there are some key differences that can help differentiate between the two.

Severity and frequency of memory problems: Age-related memory changes usually involve minor lapses, such as occasionally forgetting names or appointments. These memory lapses do not significantly interfere with daily functioning and can often be compensated for. In contrast, dementia is characterized by more pronounced and persistent memory loss that progressively worsens over time. People with dementia frequently forget important information, struggle to remember recent events, and have difficulty retaining new information.

Impact on daily life: Age-related memory changes generally do not disrupt a person's ability to perform everyday tasks and maintain independence. Forgetting a word or misplacing keys occasionally is considered normal. However, dementia impairs cognitive function to a degree that interferes with daily activities. People with dementia may struggle to manage finances, follow recipes, or complete familiar tasks that they previously handled with ease.

Progression of symptoms: Age-related memory lapses tend to remain stable or progress slowly over time. They do not typically worsen rapidly or lead to significant declines in other cognitive abilities. In dementia, memory loss is just one aspect of a broader decline in cognitive function.

Individuals may experience difficulties with language, problem-solving, decision-making, attention, and executive functions as the disease progresses.

Awareness of memory problems: Age-related memory changes are often recognized by the individual, and they may make efforts to compensate for them. They may use memory aids, develop strategies to remember information, or rely on external reminders. In dementia, individuals may be unaware of their memory loss or have difficulty recognizing the extent of their cognitive decline. They may become increasingly dependent on others to manage their daily lives.

Impact on social interactions and relationships: Age-related memory changes typically do not significantly affect a person's social interactions or relationships. They can still engage in conversations, maintain relationships, and participate in social activities. In dementia, cognitive decline can lead to difficulties in communication and social interactions. People may struggle to follow conversations, lose track of their thoughts, or have difficulty expressing themselves. These changes can result in social withdrawal and strained relationships.

Psychological and behavioral symptoms: While age-related memory changes do not typically cause significant psychological or behavioral symptoms, dementia can manifest with various non-memory-related symptoms. These may include mood swings, personality changes, irritability, agitation, anxiety, and even hallucinations or delusions. These symptoms are not typically seen in age-related memory loss.

Seeking Medical Evaluation and Diagnosis

tart by making an appointment with a healthcare professional, such as a primary care physician or geriatrician. It is essential to discuss the concerns and provide detailed information about the symptoms experienced by the individual. If possible, involve a family member or caregiver who can provide additional insights.

During the appointment, the healthcare professional will typically conduct a comprehensive medical history review. This includes discussing the individual's overall health, medications, past medical conditions, and family history of dementia or other relevant conditions. A physical examination may also be performed to rule out other potential causes for the symptoms.

The healthcare professional may administer cognitive assessments or questionnaires to evaluate memory, thinking, and other cognitive functions. These tests can provide a baseline for comparison and help identify any areas of concern. Common assessments include the Mini-Mental State Examination (MMSE) or the Montreal Cognitive Assessment (MoCA).

Blood tests may be ordered to rule out underlying medical conditions that can cause cognitive impairment or memory loss. These tests can include complete blood count (CBC), thyroid function tests, vitamin B12 level assessment, liver and kidney function tests, and more.

Imaging tests, such as magnetic resonance imaging (MRI) or computed tomography (CT) scans, may be recommended to assess the structure of the brain and rule out other possible causes for the symptoms.

Depending on the initial evaluation, the healthcare professional may refer the individual to a specialist, such as a neurologist or a geriatric psychiatrist, for further assessment and diagnosis. Specialists have expertise in diagnosing and managing dementia and related conditions.

Follow-up appointments will be scheduled to review test results, discuss the diagnosis, and develop a comprehensive management plan. The healthcare professional will explain the findings, provide information about the specific type of dementia (if diagnosed), and discuss available treatment options and support resources.

CHAPTER 3: COMMUNICATING WITH A LOVED ONE WITH DEMENTIA

Effective communication is the cornerstone of any relationship, but when a loved one has dementia, communication can become challenging and complex. This chapter explores the importance of understanding the communication difficulties faced by individuals with dementia and provides practical guidance for communicating effectively and compassionately. By improving communication skills, caregivers and family members can maintain meaningful connections and enhance the quality of life for their loved ones.

Effective Communication Strategies

Effective communication strategies are essential when interacting with individuals who have dementia. As the disease progresses, communication may become more challenging, but there are various techniques that can help improve understanding, reduce frustration, and enhance the overall quality of interactions. Be;ow are practical strategies essential in interacting with people with dementia

Maintain a calm and supportive environment: Create a calm and comfortable environment for communication. Minimize distractions, reduce noise, and ensure good lighting. Use a gentle and reassuring tone of voice to convey warmth and support.

Approach from the front: When initiating communication, approach the person from the front so that they can see you. Maintain eye contact and use non-verbal cues such as a smile or a gentle touch to establish a connection.

Use simple and clear language: Keep your language simple and straightforward. Use short sentences and one-step instructions. Avoid using complex or abstract concepts. Speak slowly and clearly, giving the person time to process and respond.

Use visual aids and gestures: Supplement verbal communication with visual aids, gestures, and visual cues. Point to objects or use hand movements to convey meaning. Visual aids such as pictures, drawings, or written notes can assist in conveying messages and promoting understanding.

Be patient and allow time for processing: Give the person with dementia ample time to process information and respond. Avoid rushing or interrupting them. Be patient and allow for pauses or breaks during the conversation.

Focus on feelings and emotions: Emphasize emotions and feelings rather than specific details or facts. Use empathetic statements to acknowledge their emotions and validate their experiences. For example, say, "I can see you're feeling sad. Is there anything I can do to help?"

Use positive and affirmative language: Frame statements and questions in a positive and affirmative manner. Offer choices when appropriate to empower the person and encourage participation. For instance, instead of saying, "Don't you remember?" you can say, "Can you tell me more about your favorite memories?"

Practice active listening: Show genuine interest and actively listen to the person. Give them your full attention and respond with empathy. Reflect back on what they say, repeat or rephrase key points to ensure understanding, and respond accordingly.

Non-verbal cues and body language: Pay attention to your own non-verbal cues and body language. Maintain an open posture, use facial expressions, and show warmth and empathy. Your non-verbal cues can convey understanding and help the person feel more at ease.

Validate and redirect: If the person expresses confusion or communicates something that doesn't make sense, avoid correcting or arguing. Instead, validate their feelings and redirect the conversation to a different topic or activity that may be more enjoyable or engaging.

Managing Challenging Behaviors

Managing challenging behaviors in individuals with dementia can be a complex task. As the disease progresses, individuals may exhibit behaviors such as agitation, aggression, wandering, or resistance to care. It's important to approach these behaviors with compassion, understanding, and appropriate strategies to ensure the safety and well-being of both the individual with dementia and their caregivers. **Identify triggers:** Pay attention to the circumstances or events that may trigger challenging behaviors. Common triggers include fatigue, hunger, pain, discomfort, unfamiliar environments, or changes in routine. Understanding the triggers can help you anticipate and prevent certain behaviors.

Maintain a structured routine: Establishing a consistent daily routine can provide a sense of familiarity and security for individuals with dementia. Stick to regular times for meals, activities, and rest to minimize confusion and anxiety.

Create a safe environment: Ensure that the environment is safe and supportive. Remove potential hazards or objects that may cause agitation or confusion. Use locks or alarms to prevent wandering if necessary. Make sure the individual has access to familiar and comforting items, such as photographs or favorite belongings.

Validate emotions and provide reassurance: Individuals with dementia may exhibit challenging behaviors as a way to express frustration, fear, or discomfort. Acknowledge their emotions, validate their feelings, and provide reassurance. Use a calm and comforting tone to let them know they are safe and cared for.

Simplify communication: Use clear and simple language when communicating. Use non-verbal cues, gestures, and visual aids to aid understanding. Break down instructions into smaller, manageable steps. Avoid arguing or correcting the person, as it can escalate their distress.

Redirect and distract: If an individual becomes agitated or fixates on a particular behavior, redirect their attention to a different activity or topic. Offer a favorite snack, engage them in a familiar hobby, or distract them with soothing music or a pleasant sensory experience.

Engage in meaningful activities: Provide opportunities for individuals to engage in activities they enjoy and that promote a sense of purpose. Activities like reminiscing, listening to music, gentle exercise, or art therapy can help reduce anxiety, improve mood, and enhance well-being.

Seek support and respite care: Caring for individuals with challenging behaviors can be emotionally and physically draining. Reach out for support from healthcare professionals, support groups, or respite care services. Taking breaks and caring for your own well-being is essential.

Consider medication and professional guidance: In some cases, medications may be prescribed to manage specific behaviors associated with dementia. Consult with healthcare professionals or specialists experienced in dementia care for appropriate assessment and guidance on medication use.

Maintain self-care: Prioritize self-care to manage stress and maintain your own well-being. Practice relaxation techniques, engage in hobbies, seek emotional support, and take breaks when needed. Remember, caring for yourself enables you to provide better care for the person with dementia.

Providing Emotional Support

Providing emotional support to individuals with dementia is crucial for their well-being and overall quality of life. The progressive nature of the disease can be challenging and overwhelming for both individuals with dementia and their caregivers. These important steps will give you a clue as to how to provide emotional support:

Show empathy and understanding: Express empathy and understanding towards the individual's emotions and experiences. Listen attentively, validate their feelings, and acknowledge their frustrations or concerns. Let them know that their emotions are valid and that you are there to support them.

Maintain a positive and calm attitude: Project a positive and calm attitude when interacting with individuals with dementia. Your demeanor and body language can influence their emotional state. Approach them with a friendly smile, use a gentle tone of voice, and maintain a relaxed posture to create a soothing environment.

Use reminiscence and validation therapy: Encourage individuals to reminisce about their past experiences, memories, and achievements. Engaging in reminiscence therapy can foster a sense of identity and self-worth. Validate their feelings and memories, even if they may not be entirely accurate. Focus on the emotions associated with their recollections.

Engage in meaningful activities: Encourage participation in activities that bring joy and a sense of purpose. Activities such as listening to music, looking at photo albums, or engaging in simple hobbies can evoke positive emotions and help individuals feel engaged and connected.

Maintain social connections: Facilitate social interactions and connections with friends, family, and community. Encourage visits from loved ones, organize social outings, or participate in group activities designed for individuals with dementia. Social engagement can alleviate feelings of isolation and boost emotional well-being.

Offer reassurance and comfort: Individuals with dementia may experience anxiety, confusion, or fear due to their cognitive challenges. Provide reassurance, comfort, and a sense of security. Use gentle touch, offer hugs, and soothing words to help them feel safe and cared for.

Be patient and flexible: Patience is key when providing emotional support to individuals with dementia. Understand that their communication abilities may change, and it may take them longer to express themselves. Be patient, give them time to respond, and avoid rushing or interrupting. Flexibility in your expectations can help reduce frustration and stress for both of you.

Encourage self-expression: Promote self-expression through various means, such as art therapy, music, or journaling. Creative outlets can serve as a channel for emotional expression, even when verbal communication becomes challenging.

Seek support for yourself: Caring for someone with dementia can be emotionally demanding. Seek support from healthcare professionals, support groups, or counseling services. Taking care of your own emotional well-being is essential to provide effective support to individuals with dementia.

Maintain a sense of humor: Use humor appropriately to lighten the mood and create moments of joy. Laughter can be a powerful tool to uplift spirits and create positive experiences. However, be sensitive to the individual's reactions and adapt your approach accordingly.

CHAPTER 4: CREATING A SUPPORTIVE ENVIRONMENT

When caring for individuals with dementia, creating a supportive environment is crucial for their well-being and quality of life. A supportive environment can help reduce confusion, minimize agitation, and promote a sense of security and comfort. This chapter explores various aspects of creating such an environment, encompassing physical, social, and emotional elements. By understanding and implementing these strategies, caregivers can provide a nurturing and safe space for individuals with dementia to thrive.

Modifying the Home for Safety and Comfort

Modifying the home environment is crucial to ensure the safety and comfort of individuals with dementia. As the disease progresses, individuals may experience cognitive and physical impairments that can increase the risk of accidents and confusion. The steps below will guide you on how to best modify your environment to best serve the need of affected.

Remove hazards and clutter: Clear the living space of any tripping hazards, such as loose rugs, clutter, or extension cords. Secure loose carpets and ensure that walkways are clear and well-lit to prevent falls.

Install safety measures: Install grab bars in bathrooms, near toilets, and in showers or tubs to provide stability and support. Use non-slip mats or adhesive strips in the bathroom to prevent slipping. Consider installing handrails in stairways and adequate lighting throughout the house to improve visibility.

Lock potentially dangerous areas: Use locks or safety devices to restrict access to potentially hazardous areas, such as basements, garages, or storage rooms. This can help prevent individuals from wandering into unsafe areas or accessing dangerous objects.

Simplify and label: Simplify the layout of the home to reduce confusion. Clearly label rooms, cabinets, and drawers using large, easy-to-read labels or pictures. Color-coding can also be helpful to differentiate areas and objects.

Ensure medication safety: Create a system to manage and store medications safely. Use pill organizers or automated dispensers to help individuals take their medications correctly and reduce the risk of medication errors. Store medications in a secure location to prevent accidental ingestion.

Implement memory aids: Use visual cues and memory aids to support daily routines and activities. For example, place visual schedules or calendars with clear instructions in easily visible locations. Use clocks with large, clear displays to help individuals understand the time of day.

Create a soothing environment: Make the home environment calming and comfortable. Use soft lighting, minimize loud noises, and create a tranquil atmosphere. Consider using soothing music or nature sounds to promote relaxation.

Ensure accessibility: Make sure that essential items are easily accessible. Keep frequently used items at waist level or within reach to minimize frustration and encourage independence. This can include clothing, toiletries, and personal items.

Provide orientation cues: Use signage or labels to provide orientation and reminders. For instance, place signs on doors to indicate the purpose of each room (e.g., "Bedroom," "Bathroom"). Use large, visible clocks to help individuals understand the time of day.

Consider technology: Explore the use of technology to enhance safety and comfort. This can include motion sensor lights, home monitoring systems, or wearable devices that can alert caregivers in case of emergencies or wandering.

Establishing Daily Routines and Structured Activities

Establishing daily routines and structured activities is beneficial for individuals with dementia as it provides a sense of stability, reduces anxiety, and promotes engagement. Routines help individuals navigate their day, provide a sense of familiarity, and enable them to maintain a sense of control.

Establish a consistent daily routine by maintaining regular times for waking up, meals, activities, and bedtime. Consistency helps individuals with dementia anticipate and understand what comes next, reducing confusion and anxiety.

Create a balance between restful and engaging activities throughout the day. Ensure that there is a mix of physical, mental, and social activities that cater to the individual's abilities and interests.

Consider the individual's preferences, interests, and abilities when planning activities. Adapt activities to their current capabilities to promote a sense of accomplishment and enjoyment.

For more complex tasks, break them down into smaller, manageable steps. This makes it easier for individuals with dementia to follow along and complete tasks successfully. Provide assistance and guidance as needed.

Use visual cues and prompts to guide individuals through their routines and activities. Visual schedules, calendars, and task lists can help reinforce the sequence of events and provide clear instructions.

While routines are important, it's essential to allow for flexibility and adjust activities based on the individual's mood, energy levels, and preferences. Be open to spontaneous activities and adapt plans accordingly.

Encourage participation in activities that are familiar and meaningful to the individual. This can include hobbies, crafts, listening to favorite music, or engaging in reminiscence activities. Familiar activities can evoke positive memories and promote a sense of connection.

This can involve spending time with loved ones, participating in group activities, or attending community events specifically designed for individuals with dementia. Social interaction helps combat isolation and promotes emotional well-being.

Create a calm and soothing environment for activities. Minimize noise, distractions, and interruptions to help individuals focus and feel more relaxed. Choose a comfortable and well-lit space for activities.

Regularly monitor the individual's response to activities and routines. Observe their engagement levels, mood, and any signs of fatigue or frustration. Be open to making adjustments and trying new activities based on their changing needs and abilities.

Promoting Independence and Autonomy

Promoting independence and autonomy is essential for individuals with dementia to maintain their sense of dignity, self-worth, and quality of life. While dementia can pose challenges to independence, there are strategies and approaches that can help individuals maintain a level of autonomy. Here are some tips for promoting independence and autonomy:

Simplify the environment: Create a safe and organized environment that supports independence. Remove clutter, minimize distractions, and arrange items in a logical and accessible manner. Label drawers and cabinets to make it easier for individuals to find what they need.

Provide cues and reminders: Use visual cues, prompts, and reminders to support independence in daily activities. For example, place labels or pictures on doors to indicate their purpose (e.g., "Bathroom" or "Bedroom"). Use clocks or timers to help individuals manage their time and routines.

Encourage self-care: Support individuals in performing activities of daily living (ADLs) independently for as long as possible. This can include tasks such as dressing, grooming, and personal hygiene. Provide assistance only when necessary and focus on promoting their abilities rather than taking over the tasks completely.

Break tasks into manageable steps: For more complex activities, break them down into smaller, achievable steps. This approach can make tasks less overwhelming and easier to complete independently. Provide guidance and support as needed, allowing individuals to take the lead in each step.

Foster decision-making: Involve individuals in decision-making whenever possible. Offer choices and options to allow them to make decisions based on their preferences and abilities. This can range from selecting clothing to participating in planning activities or outings.

Support familiar activities and hobbies: Encourage individuals to engage in familiar activities and hobbies that they enjoyed prior to dementia diagnosis. These activities can provide a sense of purpose and allow them to tap into existing skills and interests.

Focus on abilities rather than limitations: Concentrate on what individuals can do rather than their limitations. Provide opportunities for them to utilize their remaining abilities and strengths. Celebrate small achievements and offer positive reinforcement for their efforts.

Maintain familiar routines: Establish and maintain familiar routines to provide a sense of structure and continuity. Routines can help individuals anticipate and understand what comes next, promoting a sense of independence and confidence in daily activities.

Use assistive devices and technology: Explore the use of assistive devices and technology that can enhance independence. This may include items like grab bars, walking aids, medication reminders, or automated home systems that facilitate safety and independence.

Provide support and encouragement: Offer emotional support, patience, and encouragement throughout the process. Recognize and appreciate their efforts, and provide reassurance during challenging moments. Offer assistance in a respectful and empowering manner, allowing individuals to maintain their sense of dignity.

CHAPTER 5: CAREGIVING FOR A LOVED ONE WITH DEMENTIA

Caring for a loved one with dementia is a deeply rewarding yet challenging role that requires compassion, patience, and adaptability. This chapter delves into the unique aspects of caregiving for individuals with dementia, offering practical guidance, emotional support, and resources for caregivers. From understanding the progression of the disease to managing daily care tasks and prioritizing self-care, this chapter aims to empower caregivers with the knowledge and tools needed to navigate their caregiving journey.

Understanding the Role of a Caregiver

The role of a caregiver for someone with dementia is multifaceted and demanding. Caregivers play a vital role in providing physical, emotional, and practical support to individuals with dementia. This will give you a clear view on the roles of caregivers:

Personal care: Caregivers assist with the individual's personal care needs, such as bathing, dressing, grooming, and toileting. This may involve helping with hygiene routines, managing incontinence, and ensuring the individual's physical comfort.

Medication management: Caregivers often oversee medication management, ensuring that the individual takes their medications as prescribed. This includes organizing and administering medications, monitoring for any side effects, and scheduling medical appointments.

Safety and supervision: Caregivers are responsible for ensuring the safety and well-being of individuals with dementia. They may implement safety measures at home, such as removing hazards, monitoring wandering behavior, and providing supervision to prevent accidents or injuries.

Emotional support: Caregivers offer emotional support and companionship to individuals with dementia. They provide reassurance, empathy, and understanding during times of confusion, frustration, or anxiety. Building a trusting and supportive relationship is crucial for the individual's emotional well-being.

Communication and advocacy: Caregivers act as advocates for individuals with dementia, ensuring their voices are heard and their needs are met. They communicate with healthcare professionals, coordinate appointments, and relay information to ensure the best possible care and treatment.

Daily routine and activity planning: Caregivers establish and maintain daily routines to provide structure and familiarity. They plan and engage individuals in stimulating activities that promote cognitive function, social engagement, and overall well-being.

Care coordination: Caregivers often coordinate various aspects of care, including organizing home care services, managing appointments, and communicating with other family members or healthcare professionals involved in the individual's care.

Respite and self-care: Caregivers must prioritize their own well-being and self-care. They seek respite by taking breaks, seeking support from others, and maintaining their own physical and emotional health. Self-care is essential to prevent caregiver burnout and provide optimal care for the individual with dementia.

Financial and legal matters: Caregivers may assist with managing financial and legal matters on behalf of the individual with dementia. This can include budgeting, paying bills, coordinating insurance, and making legal arrangements, such as power of attorney or guardianship, when necessary.

Decision-making and end-of-life planning: Caregivers often play a role in making decisions regarding the individual's care, treatment options, and end-of-life planning. They may communicate the individual's wishes, advocate for their preferences, and consult with healthcare professionals and other family members.

Managing Caregiver Stress and Self-Care

Managing caregiver stress and practicing self-care is crucial for the well-being of caregivers themselves. Caring for someone with dementia can be demanding and emotionally challenging.

Reach out for support from family, friends, and support groups. Sharing experiences and feelings with others who understand the challenges can provide emotional relief and practical advice. Consider joining local or online support groups specifically for dementia caregivers.

Don't hesitate to accept help from others. Delegate tasks to family members, friends, or community resources. People around you may be willing to assist with specific caregiving responsibilities or provide respite care so you can have some time for yourself.

Make self-care a priority. Set aside time for activities you enjoy, such as exercising, reading, pursuing hobbies, or engaging in relaxation techniques like meditation or deep breathing exercises. Taking care of your own physical and emotional needs is vital for your well-being.

Focus on maintaining a healthy lifestyle to support your overall well-being. Eat a balanced diet, get regular exercise, and ensure you are getting enough sleep. Avoid excessive caffeine or alcohol, as they can contribute to stress and fatigue.

Take regular breaks from caregiving to recharge and rejuvenate. Arrange for respite care or ask a trusted person to take over caregiving duties for a period of time. Use this break to engage in activities that bring you joy or simply have some quiet time for yourself.

Incorporate stress reduction techniques into your daily routine. Deep breathing exercises, mindfulness meditation, yoga, or engaging in hobbies that promote relaxation can help reduce stress levels and promote a sense of calm.

Maintain social connections and relationships. Stay in touch with friends, participate in social activities, or consider joining caregiver support groups. Connecting with others can provide emotional support, reduce feelings of isolation, and offer opportunities for respite.

Be realistic about what you can accomplish as a caregiver. Understand that you have limitations, and it's okay to ask for help or seek assistance when needed. Set realistic expectations for yourself and let go of perfectionism.

Take advantage of respite care services that provide temporary relief for caregivers. Respite care allows you to have a break from caregiving responsibilities while ensuring the individual with dementia receives quality care.

Pay attention to your own physical and mental health. Schedule regular check-ups with your healthcare provider and communicate any concerns or symptoms you may be experiencing. It's important to address your own health needs.

Utilizing Respite Care and Support Services

Utilizing respite care and support services is essential for caregivers of individuals with dementia to ensure their own well-being and provide the best care possible. Respite care offers temporary relief by allowing caregivers to take breaks from their caregiving responsibilities. These are some options to consider:

In-home respite care: This service provides a trained caregiver who comes to the individual's home to provide care while the primary caregiver takes a break. In-home respite care allows the individual with dementia to remain in a familiar environment while the caregiver gets time for self-care.

Adult day programs: Adult day programs offer structured activities and social engagement for individuals with dementia during the day. Caregivers can drop off their loved ones at a community center or facility where they can participate in supervised activities while the caregiver takes a break or tends to other responsibilities.

Residential respite care: Residential respite care involves temporarily placing the individual with dementia in a residential care facility, such as an assisted living facility or nursing home, for a short period. This provides the caregiver with a more extended break, typically ranging from a few days to a few weeks.

Inpatient respite care: Some hospitals or specialized care facilities offer inpatient respite care services. This option provides temporary care for individuals with dementia in a hospital setting, particularly during times when the caregiver needs a break or is unable to provide care temporarily.

Home health care services: Home health care agencies can provide professional caregivers who come to the individual's home to provide assistance with activities of daily living, medication management, and companionship. Caregivers can arrange for scheduled visits to have time off while ensuring that their loved one receives the necessary care.

Caregiver support groups: Joining caregiver support groups, either in-person or online, allows caregivers to connect with others who are going through similar experiences. These groups provide a safe space for sharing challenges, receiving advice, and gaining emotional support from peers who understand the caregiving journey.

Counseling or therapy services: Professional counseling or therapy services can help caregivers cope with the emotional challenges and stress associated with caregiving. Therapists experienced in working with dementia caregivers can provide guidance, coping strategies, and a supportive space for caregivers to express their feelings and concerns.

Caregiver education and training programs: Many organizations offer caregiver education and training programs that provide valuable information and resources on dementia care, communication techniques, and self-care strategies. These programs can enhance caregivers' knowledge, skills, and confidence in providing care.

Respite vouchers or financial assistance: Some organizations and government programs offer respite vouchers or financial assistance specifically designed to support caregivers of individuals with dementia. These programs may provide funding or subsidies to cover the costs of respite care services, making them more accessible for caregivers.

Local community resources: Research local community resources, such as senior centers, churches, or volunteer organizations, that may offer respite care or support services for caregivers. These resources can provide additional options and support tailored to the needs of caregivers and individuals with dementia in your area.

CHAPTER 6: MEDICAL AND TREATMENT OPTIONS

Dementia is a complex neurological condition that requires a comprehensive approach to care. This chapter focuses on the medical and treatment options available for individuals with dementia, aiming to provide an understanding of the various interventions and strategies that can help manage symptoms and enhance quality of life. From pharmacological treatments to non-pharmacological interventions, this chapter explores the range of options available to healthcare professionals and caregivers in the management of dementia.

Medications and Therapies for Dementia Symptoms

There are various medications and therapies available to help manage the symptoms of dementia. It's important to note that these treatments may not reverse or cure dementia, but they can help alleviate specific symptoms and improve quality of life. Here are some commonly used medications and therapies for dementia symptoms:

Cholinesterase inhibitors: Cholinesterase inhibitors, such as donepezil, rivastigmine, and galantamine, are commonly prescribed for individuals with mild to moderate Alzheimer's disease. These medications help increase the levels of acetylcholine, a chemical messenger involved in memory and cognition, in the brain.

NMDA receptor antagonists: Memantine is an NMDA receptor antagonist that is approved for moderate to severe Alzheimer's disease. It works by regulating the activity of glutamate, a neurotransmitter involved in learning and memory processes.

Antidepressants: Antidepressant medications may be prescribed to manage symptoms of depression and anxiety, which are common in individuals with dementia. Selective serotonin reuptake inhibitors (SSRIs) and other antidepressants can help improve mood and reduce agitation or behavioral disturbances.

Antipsychotic medications: In some cases, antipsychotic medications may be prescribed to manage severe agitation, aggression, or psychosis in individuals with dementia. However, the use of antipsychotics should be carefully monitored due to potential side effects and increased risk of adverse events.

Occupational therapy: Occupational therapy focuses on helping individuals with dementia maintain their independence and engage in meaningful activities. Occupational therapists can provide strategies to compensate for cognitive impairments, improve daily functioning, and suggest modifications to the environment to enhance safety and functionality.

Cognitive stimulation therapy: Cognitive stimulation therapy involves engaging individuals with dementia in structured activities and exercises designed to enhance cognitive functioning. These activities may include puzzles, memory games, reminiscence therapy, and group discussions.

Reality orientation therapy: Reality orientation therapy aims to improve individuals' orientation to their surroundings and enhance their awareness of time, place, and personal identity. This therapy uses cues, reminders, and repetitive techniques to reinforce orientation and reduce confusion.

Reminiscence therapy: Reminiscence therapy involves discussing past experiences and memories, often using visual aids like photographs or familiar objects. This therapy helps individuals with dementia maintain a sense of identity, stimulate cognition, and provide emotional comfort.

Music therapy: Music therapy can have a positive impact on individuals with dementia, eliciting emotional responses, reducing agitation, and enhancing overall well-being. Listening to familiar music or engaging in music-related activities can stimulate memories, improve mood, and promote social interaction.

Art therapy: Art therapy involves engaging individuals in creative activities, such as painting, drawing, or crafting. This therapeutic approach can provide a means of self-expression, promote relaxation, and enhance communication skills.

Non-Pharmacological Approaches to Dementia Care

Non-pharmacological approaches to dementia care focus on providing supportive and holistic interventions that aim to enhance quality of life, reduce distressing symptoms, and promote well-being without relying on medication. These approaches can be used alongside pharmacological treatments or as standalone interventions. Here are some non-pharmacological approaches commonly used in dementia care:

Person-centered care: Person-centered care involves tailoring care to the individual's preferences, abilities, and needs. It focuses on understanding and respecting the person's unique identity, promoting autonomy, and involving them in decision-making. Person-centered care emphasizes dignity, choice, and maintaining a positive and supportive relationship with the individual.

Validation therapy: Validation therapy involves acknowledging and validating the emotions and experiences of individuals with dementia, even if they are not based in reality. Instead of trying to correct or reorient the person, validation therapy aims to empathize with their feelings, offer comfort, and create a sense of understanding and connection.

Reminiscence therapy: Reminiscence therapy involves using guided discussions, photographs, music, or other stimuli to evoke memories and encourage individuals with dementia to share and reflect on their past experiences. This therapeutic approach promotes a sense of identity, boosts self-esteem, and can facilitate social interaction.

Reality orientation therapy: Reality orientation therapy helps individuals with dementia maintain awareness of their surroundings and personal identity by providing cues, reminders, and repetitive techniques. It uses calendars, clocks, signs, and other prompts to reinforce orientation to time, place, and person.

Montessori-based activities: Montessori-based activities adapt the principles of Montessori education to engage individuals with dementia in purposeful and meaningful activities. These activities focus on sensory stimulation, fine motor skills, cognitive exercises, and engagement in familiar tasks to promote independence, engagement, and a sense of accomplishment.

Music therapy: Music therapy involves using music and rhythmic activities to elicit emotional responses, enhance mood, and stimulate cognitive function. Listening to familiar music, singing, playing instruments, or engaging in music-related activities can reduce agitation, improve communication, and promote relaxation.

Art therapy: Art therapy provides individuals with dementia an outlet for self-expression and creativity. Engaging in art activities such as painting, drawing, or sculpting can improve mood, reduce anxiety, and enhance communication. Art therapy offers a non-verbal means of communication and can be particularly beneficial for individuals with language difficulties.

Pet therapy: Interacting with trained therapy animals can provide comfort, companionship, and emotional support to individuals with dementia. Pet therapy can reduce agitation, increase social interaction, and improve overall well-being.

Sensory stimulation: Sensory stimulation involves providing individuals with dementia with sensory-rich experiences to engage their senses. This can include activities such as aromatherapy, tactile stimulation with textured objects, gentle massage, or listening to soothing sounds. Sensory stimulation can promote relaxation, reduce agitation, and increase overall sensory awareness.

Environmental modifications: Modifying the physical environment to create a dementia-friendly space can enhance safety and well-being. This includes optimizing lighting, reducing noise, using color contrast to improve visibility, and creating clear pathways to minimize confusion and promote independence.

CHAPTER 7: SUPPORTING THE ENTIRE FAMILY

Dementia not only affects the individual diagnosed but also has a profound impact on their entire family. This chapter focuses on the importance of providing support and resources to the entire family unit as they navigate the challenges of dementia. By addressing the emotional, practical, and communication needs of family members, this chapter aims to promote resilience, understanding, and well-being within the family dynamic.

Siblings and Family Dynamics

Siblings and family dynamics play a significant role in the care and support of individuals with dementia. When a family member is diagnosed with dementia, it can have a profound impact on the dynamics and relationships within the family.

Effective communication is crucial among siblings and family members when dealing with dementia. Open and honest communication allows for the sharing of information, concerns, and decision-making. It is important to maintain regular communication channels and keep everyone involved and informed about the individual's condition, treatment plans, and care needs.

Siblings may have different levels of involvement in the care of the individual with dementia. It is important to recognize and respect the different capabilities, commitments, and circumstances of each family member. Finding a balance and ensuring that responsibilities are shared fairly can help prevent resentment and foster a supportive environment.

Determine the roles and responsibilities of each family member in caregiving. Some siblings may take on primary caregiving roles, while others may provide support through financial assistance, respite care, or emotional support. Openly discuss and negotiate caregiving tasks, taking into consideration each individual's strengths, availability, and limitations.

Siblings may have different perspectives and approaches to caregiving, influenced by their personal beliefs, experiences, and relationships with the individual. It is important to respect diverse viewpoints and find common ground through open dialogue and compromise. Focus on the shared goal of providing the best care possible for the individual with dementia.

Siblings can provide emotional support to one another during the challenges of dementia caregiving. They can serve as a source of empathy, understanding, and comfort. Regular check-ins, sharing experiences, and seeking emotional support from one another can help alleviate the emotional burden and strengthen family bonds.

Conflicts may arise within the family due to differing opinions, tensions, or disagreements related to caregiving decisions or responsibilities. It is important to address conflicts constructively and seek resolution through open and respectful communication. Mediation or professional counseling services can be helpful in facilitating difficult conversations and finding solutions.

Siblings often experience significant stress and emotional strain while caring for a family member with dementia. It is crucial for siblings to prioritize self-care and seek support for their own well-being. Encourage siblings to take breaks, seek respite care, and engage in activities that promote their physical and mental health.

Talking to Children about Dementia

Talking to children about dementia requires a sensitive and age-appropriate approach. It's important to provide them with information that helps them understand the changes they may observe in their loved one and address any concerns or misconceptions they may have. Employing a sensitive and age appropriate approach requires that you tailor your explanations to the child's age and level of understanding. Use simple and clear language to explain what dementia is and how it may affect their loved one. Avoid using medical jargon or overwhelming them with too much information.

Emphasize the emotional aspect of dementia. Explain that their loved one may have trouble remembering things, may act differently, or may need extra help with daily tasks. Reassure the child that it's not their fault and that their loved one still cares about them, even if they sometimes forget or behave differently.

Encourage children to ask questions and provide honest answers. If you don't know the answer to a question, it's okay to say so and offer to find out together. Be prepared for a range of emotions and reactions from the child, including confusion, sadness, or fear.

Visual aids, such as drawings or pictures, can help illustrate and reinforce the information you're sharing. Use examples or stories that the child can relate to, such as comparing memory to a filing cabinet or explaining forgetfulness by referring to times when they may have forgotten something themselves.

Clarify that dementia is not something that can be caught or passed on to others. Explain that it is a condition that affects the brain and memory but does not mean that they or other family members will get it.

You've got to highlight that even though some things may change, there will still be routines and activities that they can enjoy with their loved one. Emphasize that the love and care within the family remain constant. Encourage them to be patient, understanding, and supportive. Teach them to offer help when needed and remind them of the positive impact they can have on their loved one's well-being.

Let children know that they can always come to you or another trusted adult with their questions or concerns. Reassure them that their feelings are valid and that they can express their emotions openly and depending on the child's age and abilities, involve them in appropriate caregiving activities. This can help them feel included, build empathy, and strengthen the bond between the child and the person with dementia.

CONCLUSION

In conclusion, dementia is a complex condition that affects individuals, families, and caregivers in profound ways. Understanding the various types of dementia, recognizing early warning signs, and seeking timely medical evaluation are crucial for effective management and care. Effective communication, managing challenging behaviors, and providing emotional support are essential components of dementia care.

Creating a safe and comfortable home environment, promoting independence and autonomy, and incorporating non-pharmacological approaches such as structured activities and therapies can significantly enhance the well-being of individuals with dementia. Additionally, building a strong support network and prioritizing caregiver self-care are vital in managing the demands and challenges of dementia caregiving.

While dementia presents unique challenges, there are strategies, resources, and interventions available to support individuals and families throughout the journey. By staying informed, seeking support, and adopting a person-centered and compassionate approach, caregivers can provide the best possible care, maintain dignity, and enhance the quality of life for individuals living with dementia.

Recap of Key Concepts

Types of dementia: Dementia refers to a group of progressive brain disorders that affect memory, thinking, behavior, and daily functioning. Common types include Alzheimer's disease, vascular dementia, and Lewy body dementia.

Early warning signs: Early warning signs of dementia may include memory loss, confusion, difficulty with language, changes in mood or behavior, impaired judgment, and withdrawal from activities.

Differentiating from age-related memory loss: Age-related memory loss is a normal part of aging and typically involves occasional forgetfulness. Dementia, on the other hand, is characterized by significant memory and cognitive decline that impacts daily functioning.

Seeking medical evaluation: If dementia is suspected, it's important to seek a medical evaluation and diagnosis. This may involve assessments by doctors, cognitive tests, brain imaging, and medical history review.

Effective communication: Communication strategies for individuals with dementia include maintaining eye contact, using clear and simple language, speaking slowly and calmly, and allowing sufficient time for responses. Non-verbal communication, such as gestures and facial expressions, can also be helpful.

Managing challenging behaviors: Challenging behaviors in dementia, such as agitation, aggression, or wandering, can be managed through a person-centered approach, maintaining routines, providing a calm environment, using validation techniques, and identifying and addressing underlying triggers.

Providing emotional support: Emotional support for individuals with dementia involves active listening, empathy, reassurance, validation of feelings, and creating a safe and supportive environment. Engaging in meaningful activities and maintaining social connections are also important for emotional well-being.

Modifying the home for safety and comfort: Modifying the home for individuals with dementia includes reducing hazards, improving lighting, using visual cues, ensuring accessibility, installing safety features like grab bars, and creating a familiar and comforting environment.

Dementia's hereditary component: While most cases of dementia are not directly inherited, certain types, such as familial Alzheimer's disease, can have a clear genetic component. However, lifestyle factors and complex gene-environment interactions also play a role in the development of dementia.

Establishing daily routines and structured activities: Daily routines and structured activities provide stability, reduce anxiety, and promote engagement for individuals with dementia. Balancing restful and stimulating activities, adapting to preferences and abilities, and providing visual cues are key strategies.

Promoting independence and autonomy: Supporting independence involves simplifying the environment, breaking tasks into manageable steps, encouraging self-care, involving the individual in decision-making, and focusing on abilities rather than limitations.

Non-pharmacological approaches: Non-pharmacological approaches to dementia care include person-centered care, validation therapy, reminiscence therapy, reality orientation therapy, music therapy, art therapy, sensory stimulation, and environmental modifications.

Building a support network: Building a support network is crucial for caregivers and involves reaching out to family and friends, joining support groups, seeking professional guidance, utilizing community resources, and prioritizing self-care.

Printed in Great Britain
by Amazon

28241740R00046